NINJA FOODI SMART XL GRILL COOKBOOK

THE COMPLETE GUIDE FOR QUICK, EASY AND DELICIOUS RECIPES I INDOOR GRILLING AND MORE.

GINA GREEN

CONTENTS

PORK RECIPES

CHICKEN RECIPES

FISH & SEAFOOD RECIPES

VEGETABLE RECIPES

SNACK & APPETIZER RECIPES

DESSERT RECIPES

INTRODUCTION

Indoor electric grills could easily be among everyone's favorite appliances of all time. Just imagine saying goodbye to the outdoors fuss and bringing the sunny grilling experience indoors not only during summer but all year round.

These kitchen gadgets come in two types: the contact grill and the open grill. The contact grill looks like a sandwich press that cooks food directly from two sides. The open grill, on the other hand, is similar to an electric griddle with ridges.

Indoor electric grills are not only popular during unfavorable weather conditions. These are also a big hit among those living in apartments and condominiums with limited space for grilling and entertaining a large group of visitors.

Using an indoor electric grill is also deemed safer and healthier as it eliminates the hazards of grilling outdoors, including burning coal, excessive smoke, and dripping fats.

With multifunctionality being a top trend in most kitchen gadgets in recent years, indoor electric grills can also do several things aside from yielding authentic char-grilled appearance, aroma, and taste in foods. Most indoor grills also function as another kitchen gadget craze—an air fryer.

One such versatile kitchen appliance is the Ninja Foodi Smart XL Grill

An Overview

What is the Ninja Foodi Smart XL Grill?

A 6-in-1 smokeless countertop grill, the Ninja Foodi Smart XL Grill can grill, air fry, bake, roast, broil and dehydrate foods. It comes with a 4-quart crisper basket and a 6-quart cooking pot. The air fry crisp function uses up to 75 percent less fat compared to deep frying.

Although this model cooks with its lid closed, only one side of food is in contact with the grill, making it an open grill type.

What are its Features and Functions?

The Ninja Foodi Smart XL Grill features a Smart Cook System and a 500-degree Cyclonic Grilling Technology for evenly cooked results.

Forget about second-guessing whether the food is undercooked or overcooked. With the Smart Cook System, a touch of a button is all it takes to get rare to well-done meat with char-grilled marks and flavors. It features a dual-sensor Foodi Smart Thermometer, four smart settings for protein, and nine doneness levels.

The 1,760-watt Ninja Foodi Smart XL Grill also boasts a smoke control system that effectively keeps smoke out of the kitchen. Coupled with a cool-air zone, it has a splatter shield and a temperature-regulating grill grate.

Perfect for family-sized meals, the XL capacity of this model translates to 50 percent more food than the original Ninja Foodi Grill version. The 9-by-12 inches grill grate can fit up to six steaks, 24 hotdogs, or a main and side dishes at the same time.

Tips for Getting Started

Using electric grills and air fryers can be intimidating if you are operating them for the first time. Fear not because we have curated a few tips that any beginner user should know. Read on and let us get you grilling and more in no time.

Always prioritize safety and set aside time for reading the user manual that comes along with the Ninja Foodie Smart XL Grill first.

Electric grills may not look like it, but they usually get hot during and after use. Practice caution and use safety tools such as tongs and oven mitts when handling the device and the food.

Place the grill on a heat-proof surface, leaving at least 5 inches of space on all sides for sufficient airflow. Also, do not place it near water to avoid electric shocks.

Allow the device to preheat for a few minutes before adding the food. Preheating will allow the grill to reach the right temperature that will give you evenly cooked and beautifully char-grilled results. Preheating also avoids extended cooking time and food from sticking to the grate.

Lightly grease the grill and basket even though they have nonstick coatings. Steer away, however, from aerosol cooking sprays as these can damage the device. We recommend getting a regular kitchen spray bottle filled with your choice of oil.

Cooking Tips & Tricks

The Ninja Foodi Smart XL Grill is practically like a convection oven. You can cook almost anything in it. You can use standard pans for baking with the air fryer function. From cakes and brownies to doughnuts and tarts--but keep an eye in case of the goods browning quickly.

You can also cook hard-boiled eggs directly in the air fryer. It would take about 15 minutes.

Try grilling vegetables such as broccoli wrapped in parchment paper. Doing so will give the vegetables the same texture from steaming, but with a hint of the charred flavor.

The air fryer is also perfect for toasting nuts. The cooking process will continue until after the nuts are unloaded from the fryer, so pull them out a bit earlier.

Frozen foods can also be cooked directly in your Ninja Foodi Smart XL Grill without thawing them first.

Say goodbye to bland and soggy leftovers—from roast chicken

and salmon to pizza and vegetables. Reheat them in the air fryer for a crispier second time (or more) around.

Less is more when it comes to oil to achieve crispiness perfection. Grease too much, and you will get soggy instead of tasty evenly cooked crispy results. Neutral oils such as canola and vegetable oils are considered best for grilling because of their high smoking point. These also do not add unwanted flavor to the food.

Save the leftover fats in the pan for later to make pan sauces and gravies.

Even with its size, make it a habit to cook in batches with your Ninja Foodi Smart XL Grill. Overcrowding food tends to obscure the hot air circulation inside, thereby affecting the crispiness and doneness of the food. Larger meats like pork chops, chicken cutlets, steaks, burgers, and fish fillets should be arranged in a single layer and not stacked one on top of the other.

Shaking the basket from time to time will also help to make sure everything inside the basket will cook and brown evenly.

Use the Foodi Smart Thermometer to check the doneness of meat accurately. Doing so not only helps to prevent overcooking but also ensures that the food is cooked enough and safe to eat.

Use oil to weigh down and glue your seasonings to the food. The air circulation inside the appliance may blow off lightweight particles such as spices while cooking. You can avoid this by mixing spices with oil before coating the food with them.

When cooking with marinated meats, let them sit on a cooling rack first to drain the excess liquids. Unlike outdoor grills, indoor grills do not drain liquid as well. So, doing this extra step will save you from cleaning marinades that dripped over your counter

Care & Maintenance Tips

With proper care and regular maintenance, your electric grill will surely last for years or even a lifetime. It is essential to clean the unit, not only to keep it running in tiptop shape but also for food safety reasons.

A sure sign that your electric grill needs some cleaning is when you start noticing smoke coming out of the machine while cooking. It signals an oil buildup. But cleaning an electric grill is so straightforward, you don't have to wait until the smoke detector alarms before taking action.

Cleaning the grill daily or after each use will avoid the accumulation of food residues in the grill. Make sure the device is turned off and unplugged, and let it cool down for a few minutes. It would be easier to clean the grate while it is still a bit hot, so take caution.

The machine itself, the basket, and the drip drawer will need a thorough cleaning. The detachable parts are dishwasher-safe, but the appliance itself is not.

The Ninja Foodi Smart XL Grill comes with a cleaning brush that you can use to get rid of the food leftovers and crumbs. Never use low quality steel items scraping food residue from the surface of the grill.

A grill brush with stainless steel handle would be a good investment for keeping your electric grill clean. You may also use a moist sponge and mild soap to remove tough stains.

Use a paper towel or soft kitchen cloth to dry the electric grill after cleaning to avoid electric shock.

Once the machine and all the detachable parts dry out completely, you may apply a bit of oil on the grill to keep it in prime condition.

Keep the lid tightly closed when the appliance is not in use to avoid minute particles like dust to accumulate in the pan. The grease may also attract bugs.

To make future cleanup easier, use a sheet of parchment paper or aluminum tin foil for items with heavy coatings. Make sure the food is heavy enough to weigh down the sheet as it may fly around due to the hot circulating air.

BREAKFAST RECIPES

1

TATER TOT EGG BAKE

Preparation Time: 10 minutes

Cooking Time: 25 minutes

Servings: 4

Ingredients:

•5 eggs

•¼ cup milk

•Salt and pepper to taste

•Cooking spray

•2 sausages, cooked and sliced

•1 cup cheddar cheese, shredded

•1 lb. frozen tater tots

Method:

1.Preheat your unit by pressing bake.

2.Set it to 390 degrees F for 3 minutes.

3.In a bowl, beat the eggs and milk.

4.Season with salt and pepper.

5.Spray a small baking pan with oil.

6.Add egg mixture to the pan.

7.Add to the unit.

8.Cook for 5 minutes.

9.Place the sausages on top of the eggs.

10. Sprinkle cheese on top.

11. Press bake and set it to 390 degrees F.

12. Cook for 20 minutes

Serving Suggestions: Garnish with chopped scallions.

Preparation & Cooking Tips: Let rest for 2 minutes before serving. Extend cooking time if eggs are not completely done.

BREAKFAST TART

Preparation Time: 10 minutes

Cooking Time: 14 minutes

Servings: 4

Ingredients:

•4 oz. cream cheese

•3 tablespoons confectioners' sugar

•¼ cup blueberry preserves

•8 oz. crescent roll dough (refrigerated)

•Cooking spray

Method:

1.Blend the cream cheese, sugar and blueberry preserves in a bowl using a hand mixer.

2.Slice the dough into 4 portions.

3.Roll out each portion until flattened.

4.Spread the cream cheese mixture on top of the dough portions.

5.Roll up the dough and seal.

6.Add these to the unit.

7.Press air crisp.

8.Preheat at 325 degrees F for 3 minutes.

9.Add the rolls to the unit.

10. Cook for 14 minutes.

Serving Suggestions: Drizzle with your favorite syrup.

Preparation & Cooking Tips: Let cool before serving.

3
___

FRENCH TOAST STICKS

Preparation Time: 10 minutes

Cooking Time: 10 minutes

Servings: 4

Ingredients:

•4 eggs

•$\frac{1}{2}$ cup milk

•$\frac{1}{4}$ cup granulated sugar

•$\frac{1}{4}$ teaspoon ground cinnamon

•$\frac{1}{4}$ teaspoon vanilla extract

•6 slices bread, sliced into strips

•Cooking spray

Method:

1.Beat the eggs and milk in a bowl.

2.Stir in the sugar, cinnamon and vanilla.

3.Dip the bread in the mixture.

4.Press air crisp.

5.Set it to 400 degrees F.

6.Preheat for 10 minutes.

7.Add the bread strips to the unit.

8. Cook for 3 to 5 minutes per side.

Serving Suggestions: Serve with maple syrup.

Preparation & Cooking Tips: Use day-old bread.

4

BREAKFAST CASSEROLE

Preparation Time: 10 minutes

Cooking Time: 10 minutes

Servings: 6

Ingredients:

• 4 eggs, beaten
• 1 lb. Italian sausage, cooked and crumbled
• 2 tablespoons heavy cream
• ½ cup cheddar cheese, shredded
• 1 cup tomatoes, chopped
• 2 teaspoons Italian seasoning

Method:

1. Combine the ingredients in a bowl.
2. Transfer to a small baking pan.
3. Select air crisp.
4. Cook at 340 degrees F for 8 to 10 minutes.

Serving Suggestions: Garnish with chopped parsley.

Preparation & Cooking Tips: Extend cooking time if eggs are not completely done.

5

QUICHE

Preparation Time: 10 minutes

Cooking Time: 15 minutes

Servings: 4

Ingredients:

•6 eggs

•¾ cup heavy cream

•Salt and pepper to taste

•1 pre-made pie crust

•1 cup cheddar cheese, shredded

Method:

1.Beat the eggs in a bowl.

2.Stir in the cream, salt and pepper.

3.Pour mixture into the pie crust.

4.Sprinkle cheese on top.

5.Press air crisp.

6.Set it to 320 degrees F.

7.Cook for 12 to 15 minutes.

Serving Suggestions: Sprinkle with chopped scallions before serving.

Preparation & Cooking Tips: You can also use homemade pie crust if you like.

6

BREAKFAST BURRITO

Preparation Time: 5 minutes

Cooking Time: 5 minutes

Servings: 2

Ingredients:

- 2 eggs, cooked scrambled
- ½ cup cheddar cheese, shredded
- ½ cup bacon, cooked crisp and crumbled
- 2 tortilla

Method:

1. Combine the eggs, cheese and bacon in a bowl.
2. Top the tortillas with the mixture.
3. Roll up the tortillas.
4. Add these to the unit.
5. Select air crisp.
6. Set it to 250 degrees F.
7. Cook for 5 minutes.

Serving Suggestions: Serve with hot sauce.

Preparation & Cooking Tips: You can also freeze the burrito and air fry when ready to serve.

7

AVOCADO TOAST

Preparation Time: 5 minutes

Cooking Time: 3 minutes

Servings: 1

Ingredients:

• 1 avocado, mashed

• 1 clove garlic, minced

• 1 teaspoon lemon juice

• Salt to taste

• 2 slices bread

• ¼ cup tomato, chopped

Method:

1. Mix the avocado, garlic, lemon juice, salt and pepper.

2. Spread mixture on top of bread slices.

3. Sprinkle tomato on top.

4. Add to the grill grate.

5. Press grill setting.

6. Grill at 350 degrees F for 2 to 3 minutes.

Serving Suggestions: Sprinkle with pepper before serving.

Preparation & Cooking Tips: Use freshly squeezed lemon juice.

8

BUTTERMILK PANCAKE

Preparation Time: 10 minutes

Cooking Time: 10 minutes

Servings: 12

Ingredients:

- •2 cups all-purpose flour
- •2 teaspoons baking powder
- •2 tablespoons sugar
- •Pinch salt
- •2 eggs, beaten
- •$\frac{1}{4}$ cup milk
- •2 cups buttermilk
- •$\frac{1}{4}$ butter, melted

Method:

1. Combine the flour, baking powder, sugar and salt.
2. Stir in the eggs and remaining ingredients.
3. Spray the air fryer tray with oil.
4. Pour the batter into the tray.
5. Select air crisp.
6. Cook at 320 degrees F for 5 minutes.

7.Flip and cook for another 5 minutes.

Serving Suggestions: Top with whipped cream.

Preparation & Cooking Tips: Flip when bubbles appear on the surface of the batter.

CHEESY BAKED EGGS

Preparation Time: 5 minutes

Cooking Time: 5 minutes

Servings: 1

Ingredients:

•2 eggs, beaten

•2 tablespoons heavy cream

•2 tablespoons cheddar cheese, shredded

•1 teaspoon Parmesan cheese, grated

•Salt and pepper to taste

Method:

1.Beat the eggs and cream in a bowl.

2.Stir in the rest of the ingredients.

3.Pour mixture into a ramekin.

4.Add the ramekin to the unit.

5.Choose air crisp setting.

6.Cook at 330 degrees F for 5 minutes.

Serving Suggestions: Garnish with chopped parsley.

Preparation & Cooking Tips: You can also add herbs to the egg mixture.

SAUSAGE PATTIES

Preparation Time: 5 minutes

Cooking Time: 10 minutes

Servings: 6-8

Ingredients:

•1 pack sausage patties

Method:

1.Add sausage patties to the air fryer tray.

2.Select air crisp.

3.Set it to 400 degrees F.

4.Cook for 5 minutes per side.

Serving Suggestions: Serve with hash browns.

Preparation & Cooking Tips: You can also make your own sausage patties if you prefer homemade.

BEEF RECIPES

11

GRILLED STEAK WITH ASPARAGUS

Preparation Time: 10 minutes
Cooking Time: 20 minutes
Servings: 5
Ingredients:
•4 strip steaks
•3 tablespoons vegetable oil, divided
•Salt and pepper to taste
•2 cups asparagus, trimmed and sliced
Method:
1.Select grill setting.
2.Choose "beef".
3.Preheat the unit by pressing "start".
4.Brush steaks with half of the oil.
5.Season with salt and pepper.
6.Coat asparagus with remaining oil.
7.Sprinkle with salt and pepper.
8.Add the steak to the grill.
9.Cook for 7 to 10 minutes per side.
10. Transfer to a plate.
11. Add the asparagus to the unit.

12. Select grill. Set it to high.

13. Serve steaks with asparagus.

Serving Suggestions: Top the steaks with a cube of butter.

Preparation & Cooking Tips: Let steaks rest for 10 minutes before slicing.

12

CHEESEBURGER

Preparation Time: 15 minutes

Cooking Time: 15 minutes

Servings: 6

Ingredients:

•2 ¼ lb. ground beef

•1 onion, chopped

•1 clove garlic, minced

•Salt and pepper to taste

•6 slices cheese

•6 burger buns

Method:

1.Combine ground beef, onion, garlic, salt and pepper.

2.Mix well.

3.Form 6 patties from the mixture.

4.Press grill setting in your unit.

5.Choose high.

6.Select beef.

7.Press start to preheat.

8.After preheating, add the patties to the unit.

9.Cook until the unit beeps.

10. Remove the burgers.

11. Add to the buns and top with cheese.

Serving Suggestions: Serve with desired condiments.

Preparation & Cooking Tips: Use 80 percent lean ground beef.

GRILLED STEAK & SALAD

Preparation Time: 10 minutes

Cooking Time: 10 minutes

Servings: 4

Ingredients:

• 4 steaks

• Salt and pepper to taste

• 4 cups lettuce, chopped

• 1 cup tomato, chopped

• 1 cup cucumber chopped

• Vinaigrette dressing

Method:

1. Press setting in your unit.

2. Set it to high.

3. Preheat for 8 minutes.

4. Season steaks with salt and pepper.

5. Add steaks to the grill.

6. Cook for 4 to 5 minutes per side.

7. In a bowl, toss lettuce, tomato and cucumber with dressing.

8. Serve steak with salad.

Serving Suggestions: Let steak rest for 5 minutes before slicing and serving.

Preparation & Cooking Tips: Use Romaine lettuce for the salad.

POT ROAST

Preparation Time: 20 minutes

Cooking Time: 3 hours and 20 minutes

Servings: 6

Ingredients:

Seasoning

•2 teaspoons thyme leaves dried

•1 teaspoon onion powder

•1 teaspoon garlic powder

•Salt and pepper to taste

•½ teaspoon red pepper flakes

Pot roast

•1 tablespoon avocado oil

•4 lb. chuck roast

•1 onion, sliced

•4 cups beef broth

•¼ cup flour

Method:

1.Mix the seasoning ingredients in a plate.

2.Coat the chuck roast with the oil.

3.Sprinkle with seasoning on all sides.

4.Preheat your unit.

5.Press grill and set it to 500 degrees F.

6.After 5 minutes, add the chuck roast to the unit.

7.Cook for 5 minutes per side.

8.Place the roast in a baking pan.

9.Pour in the broth and add the onions.

10. Choose roast setting.

11. Roast at 250 degrees for 3 hours, flipping every hour.

12. Transfer cooking liquid to a pan over medium heat.

13. Stir in flour.

14. Simmer for 10 minutes or until gravy has thickened.

Serving Suggestions: Drizzle or serve with gravy.

Preparation & Cooking Tips: Use gold potatoes.

15

STEAK & POTATOES

Preparation Time: 15 minutes

Cooking Time: 45 minutes

Servings: 4

Ingredients:

•4 potatoes

•¼ cup avocado oil

•Salt to taste

•2 steaks

•2 tablespoons steak seasoning

Method:

1.Pierce the potatoes using a fork.

2.Rub with the oil and season with salt.

3.Add to the air fryer tray.

4.Select air crisp.

5.Cook at 400 degrees F for 35 minutes or until tender.

6.Transfer to a plate and tent with foil.

7.Add the grill grate to the unit.

8.Preheat at 500 degrees F for 10 minutes.

9.Sprinkle steak fillets with steak seasoning.

10. Press grill setting.

11. Cook for 4 to 5 minutes per side.
12. Serve steaks with potatoes.

Serving Suggestions: Let rest for 5 minutes before serving.

Preparation & Cooking Tips: Use sirloin steak fillets for this recipe.

BARBECUE BEEF SHORT RIBS

Preparation Time: 20 minutes
Cooking Time: 3 hours and 15 minutes
Servings: 2
Ingredients:
•2 beef short ribs
•¾ cup beef broth
•¼ cup red wine
•¼ cup onion, diced
•½ cup barbecue sauce
Spice mixture
•1 teaspoon garlic powder
•1 teaspoon onion powder
•1 tablespoon cornstarch
•Salt and pepper to taste

Method:
1.Mix spice mixture ingredients in a bowl.
2.Season beef short ribs with this mixture.
3.Add beef ribs to a small baking pan.

4.Pour in the broth and wine.

5.Sprinkle with onion.

6.Choose roast setting.

7.Roast at 250 degrees for 3 hours.

8.Stir in barbecue sauce to the cooking liquid.

Serving Suggestions: Garnish with chopped scallions.

Preparation & Cooking Tips: Use low-sodium beef broth.

17

ITALIAN MEATBALLS

Preparation Time: 20 minutes
Cooking Time: 20 minutes
Servings: 6
Ingredients:
•1 lb. ground beef
•1 lb. ground pork
•½ onion, chopped
•3 cloves garlic, minced
•¼ cup parsley, chopped
•½ cup milk
•2 eggs, beaten
•1 teaspoon dried Italian herb seasoning
•2 tablespoons Parmesan cheese, grated
•Salt and pepper to taste
Method:
1.Mix all the ingredients in a large bowl.
2.Form meatballs from the mixture.
3.Add the meatballs to the unit.
4.Select air crisp.

5.Air fry at 425 degrees F for 20 minutes, stirring once or twice.

Serving Suggestions: Serve with pasta or brown rice.

Preparation & Cooking Tips: Use lean ground beef and lean ground pork.

18

ROAST BEEF WITH CHIMICHURRI

Preparation Time: 10 minutes
Cooking Time: 30 minutes
Servings: 6
Ingredients:
•2 lb. roast beef
•2 tablespoons olive oil
•Salt and pepper to taste
Chimichurri
•¼ cup olive oil
•½ cup cilantro
•½ cup parsley
•2 tablespoons fresh oregano, sliced
•¼ red wine vinegar
•2 cloves garlic, minced
•Salt and pepper to taste

Method:
1.Preheat your unit by pressing air crisp.
2.Press start.

3.Preheat for 4 minutes.

4.Brush roast beef with oil.

5.Season with salt and pepper.

6.Select roast function.

7.Cook at 250 degrees F for 3 hours.

8.Add all the ingredients to a food processor.

9.Pulse until smooth.

10. Serve the roast beef with chimichurri.

Serving Suggestions: Let rest steaks for 5 minutes before serving.

Preparation & Cooking Tips: You can also top the roast beef with a cube of butter.

19

GARLIC STEAK WITH CREAMY HORSERADISH

Preparation Time: 10 minutes

Cooking Time: 15 minutes

Servings: 2

Ingredients:

•2 sirloin steaks

•2 tablespoons butter, melted

•2 cloves garlic, minced

•Salt and pepper to taste

Creamy horseradish

•2 tablespoons horseradish

•1 cup sour cream

•1 teaspoon dill

•Salt and pepper to taste

Method:

1.Preheat your unit at 400 degrees F for 5 minutes.

2.Rub the butter all over the beef sirloin.

3.Sprinkle with garlic, salt and pepper.

4.Air fry for 6 minutes per side.

5.Mix the horseradish ingredients in a bowl.

6.Serve the steaks with the horseradish.

Serving Suggestions: Let steak rest for 5 minutes before serving.

Preparation & Cooking Tips: Use low-fat sour cream.

20

PARMESAN CRUSTED STEAK

Preparation Time: 5 minutes

Cooking Time: 10 minutes

Servings: 4

Ingredients:

•2 lb. flank steak

•2 tablespoons olive oil

•3 tablespoons Parmesan cheese, grated

•Salt and pepper to taste

Method:

1.Preheat your unit at 400 degrees F for 5 minutes.

2.Brush steak with oil.

3.Sprinkle with cheese, salt and pepper.

4.Select air crisp function.

Cook at 400 degrees F for 6 minutes per side.

Serving Suggestions: Serve with roasted carrots or mashed potatoes.

Preparation & Cooking Tips: Let the steak rest at room temperature for 30 minutes before seasoning.

PORK RECIPES

21

GRILLED PORK FILLET WITH VEGGIES

Preparation Time: 3 hours and 20 minutes

Cooking Time: 30 minutes

Servings: 4

Ingredients:

•3 tablespoons balsamic vinegar

•1 clove garlic, minced

•6 oz. pesto

•Salt and pepper to taste

•2 pork loin fillets

•2 tablespoons vegetable oil

•1 onion, chopped

•1 bell pepper, chopped

•1 squash, sliced

•1 zucchini, sliced into rounds

Method:

1.In a baking pan, mix vinegar, garlic, pesto, salt and pepper.

2.Add the pork.

3.Coat with the sauce.

4.Cover and refrigerate for 3 hours.

5.Select grill function.

6.Set temperature to medium.

7.Choose pork.

8.Press start.

9.In another bowl, mix the remaining ingredients.

10. Season with salt and pepper.

11. Add the vegetables and pork to the grill grate.

12. Cook until the unit beeps to signal that it's done.

13. Serve pork with veggies.

Serving Suggestions: Serve with desired condiments.

Preparation & Cooking Tips: You can also use other vegetables like potatoes or carrots.

22

FRIED PORK CUTLETS & POTATOES

Preparation Time: 20 minutes

Cooking Time: 30 minutes

Servings: 4

Ingredients:

- 1 onion, sliced
- 1 teaspoon garlic, minced
- 1 ½ lb. baby potatoes, sliced
- 1 tablespoon fresh rosemary, chopped
- Salt and pepper to taste
- 3 tablespoons honey
- 2 tablespoons mustard
- 1 cup breadcrumbs
- 4 pork cutlets

Method:

1. Toss onion, garlic, potatoes, rosemary, salt and pepper in a bowl.

2. In another bowl, mix honey and mustard.

3. Spread honey mixture on both sides of pork.

4. Dredge with breadcrumbs.

5. Add the pork to the air fryer basket.

6.Select air crisp.

7.Set it to 390 degrees F.

8.Set it to 30 minutes.

9.Press start.

10. After 10 minutes, add the potato mixture to the basket.

11. After 10 minutes, add the pork on top of the potatoes.

12. Cook for another 10 minutes, flipping once.

Serving Suggestions: Garnish with lemon wedges.

Preparation & Cooking Tips: Pork cutlets should be at least ½ inch thick.

23

PORK SANDWICH

Preparation Time: 5 hours and 30 minutes

Cooking Time: 21 minutes

Servings: 4

Ingredients:

Marinade

- 1 teaspoon onion powder
- 1 clove garlic, minced
- 1 tablespoon fresh cilantro, chopped
- 2 tablespoons soy sauce
- 2 tablespoons lime juice
- 2 teaspoons cumin
- 1 $\frac{1}{2}$ cups orange juice
- Salt and pepper to taste

Spread

- $\frac{1}{4}$ cup mayonnaise
- $\frac{1}{4}$ cup sour cream
- 1 teaspoon cumin
- 1 tablespoon lime juice

Sandwich

- 2 pork fillets

•3 bell peppers, sliced into strips and roasted

•8 slices French bread

Method:

1.Combine marinade ingredients in a bowl.

2.Add pork fillets to the bowl.

3.Cover and refrigerate for 5 hours.

4.Strain and discard marinade.

5.Add pork to the grill grate.

6.Set the unit to grill.

7.Choose high setting.

8.Set time to 11 minutes.

9.Press start.

10. Mix the spread ingredients in a bowl.

11. Spread mixture on French bread slices.

12. Add pork to the bread along with the red bell pepper.

13. Grill sandwich for 10 minutes.

Serving Suggestions: Serve with pico de gallo.

Preparation & Cooking Tips: You can also use pork tenderloin for this recipe.

24

BACON WRAPPED PORK TENDERLOIN

Preparation Time: 10 minutes
Cooking Time: 12 minutes
Servings: 4
Ingredients:
•8 slices bacon
•4 pork tenderloin fillets
•2 tablespoons vegetable oil
•Salt and pepper to taste
Method:
1.Wrap pork tenderloin with 2 bacon slices.
2.Secure with toothpicks.
3.Brush all sides with oil.
4.Season with salt and pepper.
5.Select grill function.
6.Choose high setting.
7.Set it to 12 minutes.
8.Press start.
9.After preheating the unit, add pork to the grill grate.
10. Cook for 6 minutes per side.

Serving Suggestions: Let rest for 10 minutes before serving.

Preparation & Cooking Tips: This recipe can also be used for beef tenderloin.

25

SAUSAGE & PEPPERS

Preparation Time: 10 minutes

Cooking Time: 18 minutes

Servings: 6

Ingredients:

•1 white onion, sliced into rings

•2 bell peppers, sliced

•2 tablespoons vegetable oil, divided

•Salt and pepper to taste

•6 sausages

•6 hotdog buns

Method:

1.Preheat the unit by pressing grill.

2.Set it to low.

3.Set it to 26 minutes.

4.Press start.

5.Coat the onion and bell peppers with oil.

6.Season with salt and pepper.

7.After the unit beeps, add the onion and bell pepper to the grill grate.

8.Cook for 12 minutes.

9.Transfer to a plate.

10. Add the sausages to the grill.

11. Cook for 6 minutes.

12. Add the sausages to the hotdog buns.

13. Top with the onion and pepper mixture.

Serving Suggestions: Serve with ketchup, mayo and hot sauce.

Preparation & Cooking Tips: Use whole wheat hotdog buns.

HONEY GLAZED HAM

Preparation Time: 10 minutes

Cooking Time: 50 minutes

Servings: 6

Ingredients:

• 1 cup brown sugar

• 1 cup honey

• 2 lb. ham, cooked

Method:

1. Add sugar and honey to a pan over medium low heat.
2. Simmer for 10 minutes.
3. Coat the ham with half of the sauce.
4. Place the ham inside the unit.
5. Set it to air crisp.
6. Cook at 310 degrees F for 20 minutes.
7. Brush with the remaining sauce.
8. Cook for another 20 minutes.

Serving Suggestions: Let cool before slicing and serving.

Preparation & Cooking Tips: You can also use maple syrup instead of honey.

BRATWURSTS

Preparation Time: 12 minutes

Cooking Time: 12 minutes

Servings: 4

Ingredients:

•1 pack bratwursts

Method:

1.Preheat your unit to 350 degrees F for 5 minutes.

2.Add the bratwursts to the air crisp tray.

3.Set it to air crisp.

4.Cook for 10 minutes, flipping once.

Serving Suggestions: Serve with bread or salad.

Preparation & Cooking Tips: Use a meat thermometer to find out if sausage is completely don.

APRICOT PORK CHOPS

Preparation Time: 10 minutes
Cooking Time: 10 minutes
Servings: 2

Ingredients:
•2 pork chops
•Salt and pepper to taste
•$\frac{1}{2}$ cup apricot jam
•$\frac{1}{4}$ cup water
•1 tablespoon olive oil
•1 clove garlic, minced
•1 teaspoon soy sauce

Method:
1.Season pork chops with salt and pepper.
2.Select air crisp.
3.Preheat it at 320 degrees F for 10 minutes.
4.Add pork chops to the air crisp tray.
5.Cook for 5 minutes per side.
6.In a pan over medium heat, simmer the remaining ingredients.

7.Pour the sauce over the pork chops and serve.

Serving Suggestions: Serve with rice or salad.

Preparation & Cooking Tips: Flatten the pork using a meat mallet before seasoning.

29

BREADED PORK CHOPS

Preparation Time: 10 minutes

Cooking Time: 12 minutes

Servings: 4

Ingredients:

• 4 pork chops

• Salt and pepper to taste

• 1 egg, beaten

• 1 cup bread crumbs

• 2 teaspoons sweet paprika

• 1 teaspoon onion powder

• 1 teaspoon garlic powder

• 1 teaspoon chili powder

Method:

1. Season pork chops with salt and pepper.

2. Dip pork chops in egg.

3. In a bowl, mix breadcrumbs and spices.

4. Dredge pork chops with breadcrumb mixture.

5. Select air crisp in your unit.

6. Preheat the unit for 5 minutes.

7. Add pork chops to the air crisp tray.

8.Cook at 360 degrees F for 6 minutes per side.

Serving Suggestions: Serve with fresh green salad or roasted carrots.

Preparation & Cooking Tips: Use bone-in pork chops for this recipe.

30

PORK TENDERLOIN

Preparation Time: 3 hours and 15 minutes

Cooking Time: 20 minutes

Servings: 4

Ingredients:

- 1 clove garlic, minced
- 1 teaspoon ginger, grated
- 1 tablespoon rice vinegar
- 2 tablespoons soy sauce
- 1 tablespoon vegetable oil
- 1 tablespoon dry sherry
- 1 tablespoon brown sugar
- Salt and pepper to taste
- 1 lb. pork tenderloin

Method:

1. Mix all the ingredients except pork in a bowl.
2. Once fully combined, add the pork.
3. Coat evenly with the sauce.
4. Cover and marinate for 3 hours in the refrigerator.
5. Choose air crisp function.

6.Air fry at 400 degrees F for 20 minutes, stirring once or twice.

Serving Suggestions: Let rest for 5 minutes before slicing and serving.

Preparation & Cooking Tips: You can also marinate overnight.

CHICKEN RECIPES

31

HONEY MUSTARD CHICKEN

Preparation Time: 5 minutes

Cooking Time: 30 minutes

Servings: 6

Ingredients:

•6 chicken breast fillets

•3 tablespoons vegetable oil

•Salt and pepper to taste

•1 cup honey mustard sauce

•1 cup barbecue sauce

Method:

1.Set your unit to grill.

2.Choose medium temperature.

3.Set it to 30 minutes.

4.Press start to preheat.

5.While preheating, brush both sides of chicken breast with oil.

6.Season with salt and pepper.

7.After 10 minutes, add the chicken to the grill grate.

8.Cook for 10 minutes, flipping once.

9.In a bowl, mix the honey mustard sauce and barbecue sauce.

10. Brush chicken with sauce.

11. Cook for another 10 minutes.

Serving Suggestions: Let chicken breast for 5 minutes before serving.

Preparation & Cooking Tips: You can also use thigh fillet for this recipe.

32

SPICY RANCH FRIED CHICKEN

Preparation Time: 1 hour and 20 minutes

Cooking Time: 20 minutes

Servings: 4

Ingredients:

- ½ cup buffalo sauce
- ½ cup ranch seasoning
- 4 cups buttermilk
- 2 chicken thighs
- 2 chicken breast fillets
- 2 cups all-purpose flour
- Cooking spray

Method:

1. Mix buffalo sauce and ranch seasoning in a bowl.
2. Pour into a sealable plastic bag.
3. Add buttermilk to the bag.
4. Place the chicken inside the bag.
5. Marinate in the refrigerator for 1 hour.
6. Remove from marinade.
7. Coat chicken with flour.
8. Spray with oil.

9.Select air crisp in your unit.

10. Set it to 360 degrees F and preheat for 10 minutes.

11. Add chicken to the air crisp basket.

12. Cook for 20 minutes, flipping once.

Serving Suggestions: Serve with ranch dressing.

Preparation & Cooking Tips: You can also use other chicken parts for this recipe.

33

LEMON MUSTARD CHICKEN

Preparation Time: 15 minutes

Cooking Time: 30 minutes

Servings: 6

Ingredients:

•2 tablespoons lemon juice

•¼ cup vegetable oil

•½ cup Dijon mustard

•1 tablespoon dried oregano

•3 teaspoons dried Italian seasoning

•Salt and pepper to taste

•6 chicken thighs

Method:

1.Combine all the ingredients except chicken in a bowl.

2.Mix well.

3.Brush both sides of chicken with the mixture.

4.Add chicken to the unit.

5.Choose roast setting.

6.Set temperature to 350 degrees F.

7.Select chicken.

8.Press start.

9.Transfer chicken to a plate after the unit beeps.

Serving Suggestions: Serve with fresh green salad.

Preparation & Cooking Tips: You can also use 1 whole chicken for this recipe.

34

HERB-ROASTED CHICKEN

Preparation Time: 20 minutes

Cooking Time: 5 hours

Servings: 4

Ingredients:

•1 whole chicken

•5 cloves garlic, crushed

•1 tablespoon canola oil

•¼ cup lemon juice

•¼ cup honey

•5 sprigs thyme, chopped

•2 tablespoons salt

•1 tablespoon pepper

Method:

1.Add garlic inside the chicken cavity.

2.Brush all sides of chicken with mixture of oil, lemon juice and honey.

3.Sprinkle with thyme, salt and pepper.

4.Place inside the unit.

5.Choose roast.

6.Cook at 250 degrees F for 5 hours.

Serving Suggestions: Serve with roasted vegetables.

Preparation & Cooking Tips: You can also use turkey for this recipe.

35

CHICKEN TERIYAKI

Preparation Time: 10 minutes

Cooking Time: 30 minutes

Servings: 2

Ingredients:

•2 chicken breast fillets, sliced into strips

•Salt and pepper to taste

•Cooking spray

•¼ cup teriyaki sauce

Method:

1.Season chicken strips with salt and pepper.

2.Spray with oil.

3.Add chicken strips to the grill grate.

4.Select grill setting.

5.Choose high.

6.Cook for 5 minutes per side.

7.Brush chicken with the teriyaki sauce.

8.Cook for another 10 minutes, flipping once.

Serving Suggestions: Garnish with chopped scallions and sesame seeds.

Preparation & Cooking Tips: Use low sodium teriyaki sauce.

36

CAJUN CHICKEN

Preparation Time: 20 minutes
Cooking Time: 20 minutes
Servings: 6
Ingredients:
•6 chicken drumsticks
•Olive oil
Seasoning
•1 teaspoon onion powder
•1 teaspoon paprika
•½ teaspoon dried thyme
•½ teaspoon dried basil
•½ teaspoon dried oregano
•½ teaspoon garlic powder
•½ teaspoon cayenne pepper
•Salt and pepper to taste
Method:
1.Combine seasoning ingredients in a bowl.
2.Brush chicken with oil.
3.Sprinkle both sides with seasoning.
4.Add to the air crisp basket.

5.Select air crisp setting.

6.Set to 400 degrees F.

7.Cook for 10 minutes per side.

Serving Suggestions: Garnish with fresh cilantro.

Preparation & Cooking Tips: You can also spray chicken with oil instead of brush with olive oil.

PAPRIKA CHICKEN

Preparation Time: 10 minutes

Cooking Time: 30 minutes

Servings: 6

Ingredients:

•2 lb. chicken wings

•2 tablespoons olive oil

•1 tablespoon smoked paprika

•1 teaspoon garlic powder

•Salt and pepper to taste

Method:

1.Coat chicken wings with oil.

2.Sprinkle with paprika, garlic powder, salt and pepper.

3.Add chicken wings to the air crisp tray.

4.Select air crisp.

5.Cook at 400 degrees For 15 minutes per side.

Serving Suggestions: Serve with hot sauce.

Preparation & Cooking Tips: You can also marinate the chicken for 30 minutes before air frying.

CHICKEN STUFFED WITH HERBS & CREAM CHEESE

Preparation Time: 15 minutes

Cooking Time: 15 minutes

Servings: 2

Ingredients:

•2 chicken breast fillets

•Olive oil

•2 teaspoons dried Italian seasoning

•Salt and pepper to taste

•4 oz. garlic and herb cream cheese

Method:

1.Brush chicken with oil.

2.Sprinkle with Italian seasoning, salt and pepper.

3.Top with garlic and herb cream cheese.

4.Roll up the chicken.

5.Place on the air crisp tray.

6.Air fry at 370 degrees F for 7 minutes per side.

Serving Suggestions: Serve with fresh green salad.

Preparation & Cooking Tips: You can also freeze the stuffed chicken and air fry when ready to serve.

HONEY SRIRACHA CHICKEN

Preparation Time: 20 minutes
Cooking Time: 15 minutes
Servings: 4

Ingredients:
•2 lb. chicken tenders
•2 tablespoons olive oil
•Salt and pepper to taste
Honey sriracha sauce
•½ cup honey
•2 teaspoons sriracha
•1 tablespoon garlic powder
•2 tablespoons soy sauce
•2 teaspoons cornstarch

Method:
1.Brush chicken with oil.
2.Season with salt and pepper.
3.Place inside the unit, on the air crisp basket.
4.Select air crisp setting.
5.Air fry at 370 degrees F for 5 minutes per side.
6.Mix the sauce ingredients in a bowl.

7.Dip the chicken in the sauce.

8.Place the chicken back to the air crisp tray.

9.Cook at 400 degrees F for 5 minutes.

Serving Suggestions: Garnish with chopped chives.

Preparation & Cooking Tips: You can also use chicken breast strips for this recipe.

40

BARBECUE CHICKEN

Preparation Time: 10 minutes

Cooking Time: 30 minutes

Servings: 4

Ingredients:

•4 chicken breast fillets

•2 tablespoons oil

•Salt and pepper to taste

•1 cup barbecue sauce

Method:

1.Choose grill setting.

2.Set temperature to medium.

3.Set it to 30 minutes.

4.Press start to preheat.

5.Brush chicken breast with oil.

6.Season with salt and pepper.

7.After 5 minutes, add chicken to the grill grate.

8.Cook chicken for 10 minutes per side.

9.Dip chicken in barbecue sauce and cook for another 5 minutes.

. . .

Serving Suggestions: Serve with remaining barbecue sauce.

Preparation & Cooking Tips: You can also serve with other grilled vegetables.

FISH & SEAFOOD RECIPES

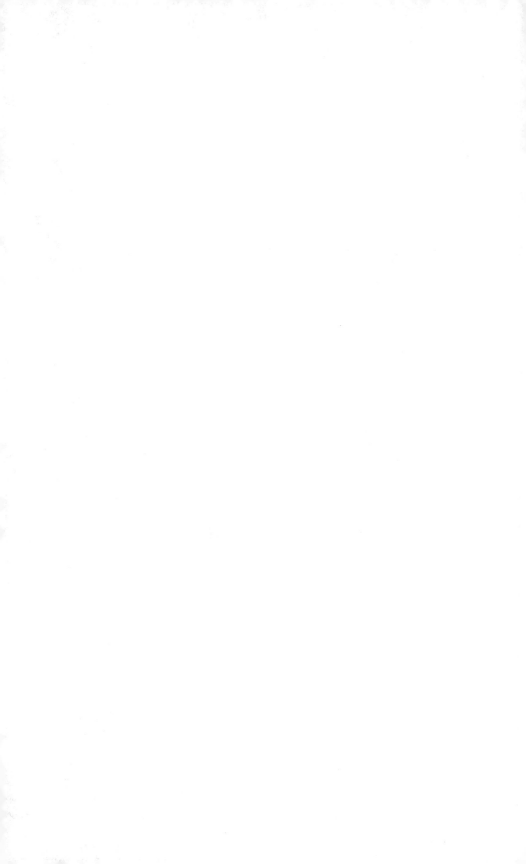

41

MAHI & SALSA

Preparation Time: 15 minutes
Cooking Time: 12 minutes
Servings: 4
Ingredients:
•4 mahi fillets
•4 tablespoons vegetable oil
•Salt and pepper to taste
Basting
•¼ cup honey
•3 tablespoons lime juice
•2 tablespoons creole seasoning
•1 tablespoon cilantro, chopped
Salsa
•1 teaspoon cumin
•¼ cup lime juice
•1 tablespoon cilantro, chopped
•1 cup pineapple chunks
•1 red bell pepper, chopped
•1 onion, chopped
•1 jalapeño pepper, chopped

Method:

1.Coat fish with oil.

2.Season with salt and pepper.

3.In a bowl, mix basting ingredients.

4.Set your unit to grill.

5.Set temperature to max and time to 15 minutes.

6.Press start.

7.After unit beeps, add fish to the grill.

8.Brush the top with the basting sauce.

9.Cook for 6 minutes.

10. Flip and brush the other side with the sauce.

11. Cook for another 6 minutes.

12. In another bowl, mix the salsa ingredients.

13. Serve fish with salsa.

Serving Suggestions: Garnish with cucumber and tomato slices.

Preparation & Cooking Tips: You can also grill pineapple rings and slice to be used for the salsa.

42

SHRIMP TACOS

Preparation Time: 20 minutes

Cooking Time: 5 minutes

Servings: 6

Ingredients:

•1 lb. shrimp, peeled and deveined

•2 tablespoons vegetable oil

•2 tablespoons Cajun seasoning

•Salt and pepper to taste

•6 corn tortillas

Toppings

•Pico de gallo

•Avocado, sliced

•Cabbage, shredded

•Lime wedges

Method:

1.Select grill setting.

2.Set temperature to max.

3.Enter 3 minutes.

4.Press start to preheat.

5.Coat shrimp with oil.

6.Season with Cajun seasoning, salt and pepper.

7.After unit beeps, add the shrimp to the grill grate.

8.Select grill.

9.Choose high temperature.

10. Set time to 2 minutes.

11. Top the tortillas with toppings and grilled shrimp.

12. Roll up and serve.

Serving Suggestions: Sprinkle with chopped cilantro.

Preparation & Cooking Tips: You can use frozen shrimp for this recipe but extend cooking time for another minute.

43

SALMON WITH LEMON & DILL

Preparation Time: 15 minutes
Cooking Time: 20 minutes
Servings: 6

Ingredients:
•6 salmon fillets
•1 tablespoon vegetable oil
•Salt and pepper to taste
•¼ cup mayonnaise
•2 tablespoons Dijon mustard
•4 tablespoons lemon juice
•2 tablespoons dill, chopped
•4 teaspoons garlic, minced

Method:
1.Choose grill setting in your unit.
2.Set temperature to max.
3.Select fish.
4.Press start to preheat.
5.Brush both sides of salmon with oil.
6.Season with salt and pepper.
7.Add salmon to the grill grate.

8. In a bowl, mix the remaining ingredients.

9. Brush mixture on top side of salmon.

10. Top with lemon slices.

11. Close the unit.

12. Wait for it to beep to signal that cooking is complete.

Serving Suggestions: Let rest for 3 minutes before serving.

Preparation & Cooking Tips: You can also use white fish fillet for this recipe.

44

LEMON MUSTARD FISH

Preparation Time: 10 minutes

Cooking Time: 10 minutes

Servings: 2

Ingredients:

- 2 tablespoons lemon juice
- 1 tablespoon Dijon mustard
- 2 tablespoons olive oil
- 2 cloves garlic, minced
- $\frac{1}{2}$ teaspoon ground thyme
- Salt and pepper to taste
- 2 fish fillets

Method:

1. Combine all the ingredients in a bowl.
2. Spread mixture on top side of the fish.
3. Add salmon to the air crisp tray.
4. Select air crisp in your unit.
5. Air fry at 400 degrees F for 7 to 10 minutes.

Serving Suggestions: Garnish with lemon wedges.

Preparation & Cooking Tips: You can use frozen fish for

this recipe but make sure that you thaw first before seasoning and air frying.

45

SHRIMP BANG

Preparation Time: 10 minutes

Cooking Time: 10 minutes

Servings: 4

Ingredients:

•1 lb. large shrimp, peeled and deveined

•¼ cup flour

•2 eggs, beaten

•2 cups breadcrumbs

Sauce

•¼ cup mayonnaise

•2 tablespoons sweet chili sauce

•2 teaspoons sriracha sauce

•1 tablespoon honey

•1 teaspoon rice vinegar

Method:

1.Coat the shrimp with flour.

2.Dip in egg and then dredge with breadcrumbs.

3.Select air crisp setting.

4.Preheat at 250 degrees F for 7 minutes.

5.Add the breaded shrimp to the air crisp tray.

6.Cook at 350 degrees F for 5 minutes per side.

7.Mix the sauce ingredients.

8.Serve shrimp with sauce.

Serving Suggestions: Sprinkle with chopped chives before serving.

Preparation & Cooking Tips: You can also dip the shrimp in the sauce right away before serving.

46

FRIED CLAMS

Preparation Time: 5 minutes

Cooking Time: 5 minutes

Servings: 4

Ingredients:

•1 pack frozen clams

Method:

1.Preheat your unit to 400 degrees F for 5 minutes.

2.Add clams to the air crisp tray.

3.Cook for 5 minutes.

4.Check to see if they are done. If not, cook for another 3 to 5 minutes.

Serving Suggestions: Garnish with lemon wedges.

Preparation & Cooking Tips: You can season clams with dried herbs if you like.

Shrimp Tempura

Preparation Time: 5 minutes

Cooking Time: 10 minutes

Servings: 6

Ingredients:

•1 pack frozen shrimp tempura

Method:

1.Preheat the air fryer to 390 degrees F for 5 minutes.

2.Arrange the frozen tempura on a single layer on your air crisp basket.

3.Cook the shrimp for 5 minutes per side.

Serving Suggestions: Serve with mirin or soy sauce.

Preparation & Cooking Tips: Make sure that there are no shrimp overlapping.

GARLIC BUTTER SHRIMP

Preparation Time: 10 minutes

Cooking Time: 5 minutes

Servings: 4

Ingredients:

Garlic butter sauce

• 2 cloves garlic, minced

• ½ cup butter, melted

• 1 teaspoon dried parsley

• Salt and pepper to taste

Shrimp

• 1 lb. shrimp, peeled and deveined

Method:

1. Combine garlic butter sauce ingredients in a bowl.
2. Coat the shrimp with this mixture.
3. Add to the air crisp tray.
4. Set it to air crisp.
5. Air fry at 400 degrees F for 5 minutes.

Serving Suggestions: Sprinkle with chopped chives.

Preparation & Cooking Tips: You can also serve shrimp with the remaining garlic butter sauce.

SWORDFISH FILLET WITH SALSA

Preparation Time: 10 minutes
Cooking Time: 10 minutes
Servings: 4
Ingredients:
•4 swordfish fillets
•1 tablespoon vegetable oil
•Salt and pepper to taste
Salsa
•1 onion, chopped
•2 mangoes, diced
•½ cup cilantro, chopped
•2 tablespoons lime juice
Method:
1.Brush fish with oil.
2.Season both sides with salt and pepper.
3.Marinate for 5 minutes.
4.Place in the air crisp tray.
5.Select air crisp.
6.Cook at 400 degrees F for 5 minutes per side.

7.Mix the salsa ingredients in a bowl.

Top the fish with the salsa and serve.

Serving Suggestions: Sprinkle chopped cilantro on top.

Preparation & Cooking Tips: Use freshly squeezed lime juice.

49

TUNA BURGER

Preparation Time: 10 minutes
Cooking Time: 10 minutes
Servings: 4
Ingredients:
•Cooking spray
Tuna patties
•6 oz. tuna flakes
•1 tablespoon lemon juice
•1 teaspoon lemon zest
•1 teaspoon Dijon mustard
•1 egg, beaten
•1 tablespoon Italian seasoning
•½ cup breadcrumbs
Burger
•4 burger buns
•Lettuce leaves
•1 tomato, sliced
Method:
1.Mix tuna patty ingredients in a bowl.
2.Form 4 patties from the mixture.

3.Spray the patties with oil.

4.Place these in the air crisp tray.

5.Choose air crisp setting.

6.Air fry 360 degrees F for 5 minutes per side.

7.Serve in burger buns with tomato and lettuce.

Serving Suggestions: Serve with desired condiments.

Preparation & Cooking Tips: You can also make the patties in advance, freeze and the air fry when ready to serve.

VEGETABLE RECIPES

50

MAPLE GLAZED SQUASH

Preparation Time: 10 minutes

Cooking Time: 40 minutes

Servings: 8

Ingredients:

•2 butternut squash, sliced

•1 tablespoon vegetable oil

•Salt and pepper to taste

•2 tablespoons butter

•4 tablespoons maple syrup

•4 tablespoons brown sugar

Method:

1.Coat butternut squash with oil.

2.Season with salt and pepper.

3.Select roast setting.

4.Set it to 375 degrees F for 45 minutes.

5.Press start to preheat.

6.After the unit beeps, add the butternut squash to the grill grate.

7.Cook the squash for 20 minutes.

8.While waiting, combine the remaining ingredients.

9.Dip the squash in the sauce and return to the grill.

10. Cook for another 15 minutes.

11. Flip and cook for 5 more minutes.

Serving Suggestions: Garnish with chopped fresh thyme.

Preparation & Cooking Tips: You can also use this recipe for carrots.

51

VEGGIE FLATBREAD

Preparation Time: 30 minutes

Cooking Time: 10 minutes

Servings: 6

Ingredients:

- 1 teaspoon olive oil
- 1 lb. pizza dough
- 1 tablespoon olive oil
- ¼ cup zucchini, sliced thinly
- ¼ cup squash, sliced thinly
- 1 teaspoon garlic, minced
- ½ cup Parmesan cheese, grated
- ½ teaspoon red pepper flakes

Method:

1. Coat the dough with 1 teaspoon olive oil.
2. Let sit at room temperature for 15 minutes.
3. Select grill setting.
4. Set it to high for 10 minutes.
5. Press start to preheat.
6. Add pizza dough to the grill grate.
7. Cook for 3 minutes.

8.Flip and cook for another 1 minute.

9.Take the flatbread out of the unit.

10. Brush the top with the remaining olive oil.

11. Add the remaining ingredients on top.

12. Place inside the unit.

13. Cook for 5 minutes.

14. Let cool, slice and serve.

Serving Suggestions: Garnish with fresh basil.

Preparation & Cooking Tips: You can also use pizza crust for this recipe.

52

MEXICAN CORN

Preparation Time: 15 minutes

Cooking Time: 12 minutes

Servings: 6

Ingredients:

•6 ears corn

•3 tablespoons canola oil

•Salt and pepper to taste

•1 ¼ cups Cotija cheese, crumbled

•2 teaspoons onion powder

•2 teaspoons garlic powder

•½ cup sour cream

•½ cup mayonnaise

•2 tablespoons lime juice

Method:

1.Select grill function.

2.Set temperature to max.

3.Set it to 12 minutes.

4.Press start to preheat.

5.Brush the corn ears with oil.

6.Sprinkle all sides with salt and pepper.

7.Place on the grill grate and cook for 6 minutes per side.

8.Mix the remaining ingredients in a bowl.

9.Cover the corn with the mixture and serve.

Serving Suggestions: Garnish with fresh cilantro.

Preparation & Cooking Tips: Use low-fat sour cream.

53

ROASTED POTATOES & ASPARAGUS

Preparation Time: 10 minutes

Cooking Time: 10 minutes

Servings: 4

Ingredients:

- 1 lb. asparagus, trimmed and sliced
- 1 tablespoon olive oil
- 2 stalks scallions, chopped
- 4 potatoes, diced and boiled
- 1 teaspoon dried dill
- Salt and pepper to taste

Method:

1. Coat asparagus with oil.
2. Sprinkle it with scallions.
3. Place in the air fryer tray.
4. Select air crisp.
5. Cook at 350 degrees F for 5 minutes.
6. Transfer to a bowl.
7. Stir in the rest of the ingredients.

Serving Suggestions: Garnish with lemon wedges.

Preparation & Cooking Tips: You can also use fresh chopped dill for this recipe.

LEMON PEPPER BRUSSELS SPROUTS

Preparation Time: 10 minutes

Cooking Time: 10 minutes

Servings: 4

Ingredients:

•1 lb. Brussels sprouts, sliced

•tablespoons olive oil

•2 teaspoons lemon pepper seasoning

•Salt to taste

Method:

1.Coat the Brussels sprouts with oil.

2.Season with lemon pepper seasoning and salt.

3.Spread these on the air crisp tray.

4.Select broil setting.

5.Cook at 350 degrees F for 5 minutes.

Serving Suggestions: Serve with mayo-based dip.

Preparation & Cooking Tips: You can also use cauliflower for this recipe.

BALSAMIC ROASTED TOMATOES WITH HERBS

Preparation Time: 5 minutes

Cooking Time: 5 minutes

Servings: 4

Ingredients:

• 1 lb. tomatoes, sliced into quarters

• ½ cup balsamic vinegar

• 1 teaspoon Italian seasoning

Method:

1. Toss tomatoes in balsamic vinegar.

2. Sprinkle with Italian seasoning.

3. Add to the air crisp tray.

4. Select air crisp.

5. Cook at 350 degrees F for 5 minutes.

Serving Suggestions: Sprinkle with chopped herbs.

Preparation & Cooking Tips: You can also stir in cucumber slices into the mix after air frying.

Squash with Thyme & Sage

Preparation Time: 10 minutes

Cooking Time: 15 minutes

Servings: 4

Ingredients:

•2 lb. butternut squash, sliced into cubes

•1 tablespoon olive oil

•Salt to taste

•1 teaspoon fresh thyme, chopped

•1 tablespoon fresh sage, chopped

Method:

1.Preheat your air fryer to 390 degrees F.

2.Coat the squash cubes with oil.

3.Season with salt, pepper, thyme and sage.

4.Add to the air crisp tray.

5.Cook for 10 minutes.

6.Flip and cook for another 5 minutes.

Serving Suggestions: Sprinkle with pepper.

Preparation & Cooking Tips: Check to see if squash is tender enough. If not, cook for a few more minutes.

GARLIC CARROTS

Preparation Time: 10 minutes

Cooking Time: 10 minutes

Servings: 4

Ingredients:

•1 lb. carrots, diced

•2 tablespoons olive oil

•2 teaspoons garlic powder

•Salt and pepper to taste

Method:

1.Toss the carrot cubes in olive oil.

2.Season with garlic powder, salt and pepper.

3.Coat evenly.

4.Spread carrots in the air crisp tray.

5.Cook at 390 degrees F for 10 minutes, stirring once.

Serving Suggestions: Sprinkle with chopped parsley.

Preparation & Cooking Tips: You can also use minced garlic instead of garlic powder.

ZUCCHINI FRITTERS

Preparation Time: 10 minutes

Cooking Time: 7 minutes

Servings: 2

Ingredients:

•2 cups zucchini, grated

•1 clove garlic, minced

•1 egg, beaten

•¼ cup Parmesan cheese, grated

•½ cup breadcrumbs

•Salt and pepper to taste

•Cooking spray

Method:

1.Combine the ingredients in a bowl.

2.Form patties from the mixture.

3.Add these to the air crisp tray.

4.Spray with oil.

5.Select air crisp.

6.Cook at 390 degrees F for 7 minutes.

Serving Suggestions: Garnish with chopped parsley.

Preparation & Cooking Tips: Add the breadcrumbs last in the mixture.

58

BUFFALO CAULIFLOWER

Preparation Time: 15 minutes

Cooking Time: 15 minutes

Servings: 4

Ingredients:

•4 cups cauliflower florets

•½ cup buffalo sauce

•2 tablespoons olive oil

•Salt to taste

•1 teaspoon garlic powder

Method:

1.Coat the cauliflower with buffalo sauce and olive oil.

2.Season with salt and garlic powder.

3.Spread in the air crisp tray.

4.Choose air crisp setting.

5.Cook at 375 degrees F for 15 minutes, stirring twice.

Serving Suggestions: Serve with additional buffalo sauce.

Preparation & Cooking Tips: You can also drizzle with hot sauce.

SNACK & APPETIZER RECIPES

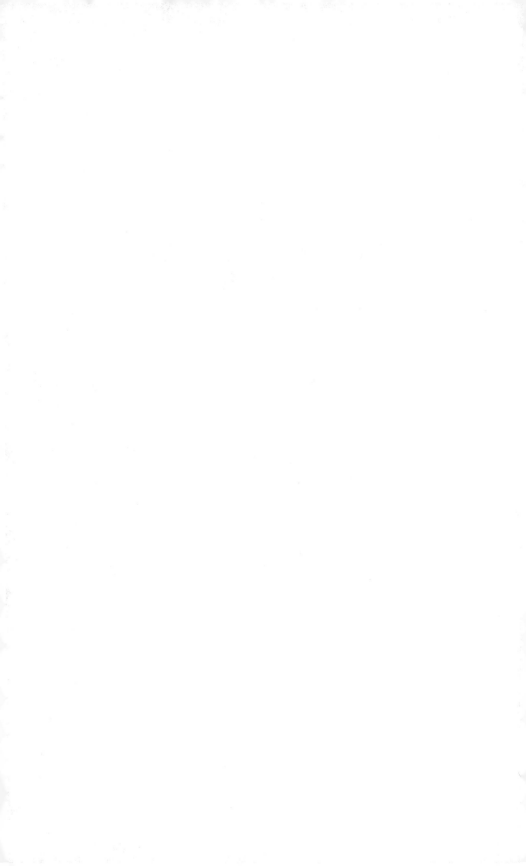

TACO CUPS

Preparation Time: 20 minutes

Cooking Time: 10 minutes

Servings: 8

Ingredients:

• 12 wonton wrappers

• 1 lb. ground beef, cooked

• ½ cup tomatoes, chopped

• 2 tablespoons taco seasoning

• 1 cup cheddar cheese, shredded

Method:

1. Press the wrappers onto cups of a muffin pan.

2. Place inside the unit.

3. Air fry at 400 degrees F for 5 minutes.

4. Take it out of the unit.

5. Top with the ground beef and tomatoes.

6. Sprinkle with the taco seasoning and cheese.

7. Air fry for another 5 minutes.

Serving Suggestions: Serve with guacamole, salsa and sour cream.

Preparation & Cooking Tips: Use lean ground beef.

CORN FRITTERS

Preparation Time: 10 minutes

Cooking Time: 8 minutes

Servings: 6

Ingredients:

• ½ cup all-purpose flour

• 1 ½ cup corn kernels

• 1 teaspoon sugar

• ¼ cup milk

• 1 egg, beaten

• 2 stalks green onion, chopped

• ½ cup cheddar cheese, shredded

• Salt and pepper to taste

• Cooking spray

Method:

1. Combine all the ingredients in a bowl.

2. Drop 2 to 3 tablespoons of the mixture onto the air crisp tray.

3. Spray with oil.

4. Select air crisp function.

5.Air fry at 350 degrees F for 3 minutes.

6.Flip and air fry for another 5 minutes.

Serving Suggestions: Serve with sour cream.

Preparation & Cooking Tips: You can also use almond milk for this recipe.

61

GARLIC BREAD

Preparation Time: 10 minutes
Cooking Time: 5 minutes
Servings: 4

Ingredients:
• 4 cloves roasted garlic, chopped
• ½ cup butter, melted
• 1 tablespoon fresh parsley, chopped
• 1 loaf Italian bread
• Salt to taste

Method:
1. Mix the garlic, butter and parsley in a bowl.
2. Spread the mixture on the bread slices.
3. Place the bread inside the unit.
4. Choose air crisp setting.
5. Cook at 400 degrees F for 3 minutes.

Serving Suggestions: Let cool for 2 minutes before serving.

Preparation & Cooking Tips: You can also use French bread for this recipe.

62

PEPPERONI PIZZA

Preparation Time: 15 minutes
Cooking Time: 7 minutes
Servings: 6

Ingredients:
- 1 lb. pizza dough
- Cooking spray
- 1 cup pizza sauce
- ½ cup mozzarella cheese
- ¼ cup pepperoni slices

Method:
1. Spray the dough with oil.
2. Knead for 5 to 10 minutes.
3. Roll onto a small pizza pan.
4. Spread pizza sauce on top.
5. Sprinkle cheese and top with pepperoni slices.
6. Add the pizza pan to the unit.
7. Select air crisp setting.
8. Air fry at 375 degrees F for 7 minutes.

Serving Suggestions: Garnish with herbs.

Preparation & Cooking Tips: You can also use frozen pizza crust to reduce preparation time.

63

GOAT CHEESE TARTS WITH TOMATOES

Preparation Time: 10 minutes
Cooking Time: 8 minutes
Servings: 8

Ingredients:

•Cooking spray
•1 tablespoon honey
•1 teaspoon dried Italian seasoning
•½ cup goat cheese, crumbled
•1 pack crescent rounds
•2 tomatoes, chopped
•2 tablespoons olive oil

Method:

1.Spray your muffin pan with oil.
2.In a bowl, mix the honey, Italian seasoning and goat cheese.
3.Slice the dough into 8 portions.
4.Press the dough onto the cups of your muffin pan.
5.Coat the tomatoes with oil.
6.Place tomatoes on top of the dough.
7.Top with the goat cheese mixture.
8.Place inside the unit.

9.Set it to bake.

10. Cook at 330 degrees F for 8 minutes.

Serving Suggestions: Sprinkle with herbs on top.

Preparation & Cooking Tips: Extend cooking time until crust is golden.

MOZZARELLA BITES

Preparation Time: 20 minutes

Cooking Time: 8 minutes

Servings: 12

Ingredients:

• 12 mozzarella strips

• ¼ cup butter, melted

• 1 cup breadcrumbs

Method:

1. Dip mozzarella strips in butter.

2. Dredge with breadcrumbs.

3. Add the mozzarella strips to the air crisp tray.

4. Select air crisp setting.

5. Cook at 320 degrees F for 8 minutes, flipping once.

Serving Suggestions: Serve with marinara dip.

Preparation & Cooking Tips: You can also make the mozzarella bites ahead of time and freeze. Air fry when ready to serve.

SPICY CHICKPEAS

Preparation Time: 5 minutes
Cooking Time: 10 minutes
Servings: 4
Ingredients:
•15 oz. canned chickpeas, rinsed and drained
•1 tablespoon olive oil
•1 teaspoon chili powder
•1 teaspoon ground cumin
•½ teaspoon cayenne pepper
•Salt to taste
Method:
1.Coat the chickpeas with oil.
2.Season with chili powder, cumin, cayenne pepper and salt.
3.Add to the air crisp tray.
4.Press air crisp function.
5.Cook at 390 degrees F for 10 minutes, stirring once or twice.
Serving Suggestions: Let cool before serving or storing.
Preparation & Cooking Tips: Do not overcrowd the air crisp tray.

NAAN PIZZA

Preparation Time: 5 minutes

Cooking Time: 5 minutes

Servings: 1

Ingredients:

•Cooking spray

•1 naan bread

•¼ cup pesto

•½ cup baby spinach, cooked

•½ cup cherry tomatoes, sliced in half

•1 cup mozzarella cheese

Method:

1.Spray your air crisp tray with oil.

2.Spread pesto on top of the naan bread.

3.Top with spinach and tomatoes.

4.Sprinkle cheese on top.

5.Add naan pizza to the air crisp tray.

6.Choose air crisp setting.

7.Cook at 350 degrees F for 7 minutes.

Serving Suggestions: Garnish with fresh herbs.

Preparation & Cooking Tips: You can also use pizza sauce instead of pesto if you like.

67

CHILI CHEESY FRIES

Preparation Time: 5 minutes

Cooking Time: 14 minutes

Servings: 6

Ingredients:

•1 package frozen French fry

•Salt and pepper to taste

•15 oz. chili

•½ cup cheese, shredded

Method:

1.Add French fries to the air crisp tray.

2.Select air crisp setting.

3.Set temperature to 400 degrees.

4.Set time to 15 minutes.

5.Flip French fries halfway through cooking.

6.In a pan over medium heat, add the chili and cheese.

7.Spread mixture over the fries.

Serving Suggestions: Top with sour cream before serving.

Preparation & Cooking Tips: You can also use homemade fries for this recipe.

68

BAKED POTATO ROUNDS

Preparation Time: 10 minutes

Cooking Time: 18 minutes

Servings: 8

Ingredients:

•2 large potatoes, sliced into thick rounds

•Cooking spray

•Salt and pepper to taste

•1 cup cheese, shredded

•4 bacon slices, cooked crisp and crumbled

Method:

1.Add the potatoes to the air crisp tray.

2.Spray the top part with oil.

3.Sprinkle with salt and pepper.

4.Select air crisp setting.

5.Air fry the potatoes at 370 degrees F for 7 to 8 minutes per side.

6.Remove from the unit.

7.Top each potato with cheese and bacon bits.

8.Air fry for another 2 minutes or until cheese has melted.

Serving Suggestions: Serve with sour cream.
Preparation & Cooking Tips: Use Russet potatoes.

DESSERT RECIPES

69

APPLE TART

Preparation Time: 20 minutes

Cooking Time: 12 minutes

Servings: 8

Ingredients:

• 8 teaspoons brown sugar

• 4 tablespoons granulated sugar

• 2 teaspoons ground cinnamon

• 1 ½ teaspoons lemon juice

• 4 apples, sliced thinly

• Pinch salt

• 1 package biscuit dough

• Cooking spray

Method:

1. Mix sugars and cinnamon in a bowl.

2. Take 1 ½ tablespoons of this mixture and transfer to another bowl.

3. Stir in lemon juice, apples and salt.

4. Mix until fully combined.

5. Roll out the dough and separate into smaller pieces.

6. Top each piece with apple mixture.

7.Top with another piece and press the edges to seal.

8.Add to the grill grate.

9.Choose grill setting.

10. Set it to low.

11. Set time to 9 minutes.

12. Press start to preheat.

13. Grill for 6 minutes per side.

Serving Suggestions: Serve with vanilla ice cream.

Preparation & Cooking Tips: Use pre-made biscuit dough.

70

APPLE CAKE

Preparation Time: 15 minutes

Cooking Time: 20 minutes

Servings: 6

Ingredients:

•1 cup brown sugar

•3 eggs, beaten

•1 cup apples, diced

•1 cup all-purpose flour

•Cooking spray

Method:

1.Mix eggs and sugar in a bowl.

2.Fold in the flour and mix well.

3.Stir in the apples.

4.Spray your pie pan with oil.

5.Pour the mixture into the pie pan.

6.Place inside the unit.

7.Set it to bake.

8.Cook at 320 degrees F for 15 to 20 minutes.

Serving Suggestions: Drizzle with maple syrup.

Preparation & Cooking Tips: Extend cooking time if pie is not fully cooked.

71

BUTTER CAKE

Preparation Time: 10 minutes

Cooking Time: 12 minutes

Servings: 6

Ingredients:

•14 oz. cookie butter

•3 eggs, beaten

•¼ cup granulated sugar

•Cooking spray

Method:

1.Microwave cookie butter for 90 seconds, stirring every 30 seconds.

2.In a bowl, add the cookie butter, eggs and sugar.

3.Spray a small baking pan with oil.

4.Pour the batter onto the baking pan.

5.Air fry at 320 degrees F for 10 minutes.

Serving Suggestions: Let cool before slicing and serving.

Preparation & Cooking Tips: Extend cooking time if not fully done.

• • •

Chocolate Chip Cookies

Preparation Time: 5 minutes

Cooking Time: 15 minutes

Servings: 12

Ingredients:

•15 oz. yellow cake mix

•¼ cup butter, melted

•2 eggs, beaten

•1 cup chocolate chips

Method:

1.Combine all the ingredients in a bowl.

2.Form cookies from the mixture.

3.Add the cookies to the air crisp tray.

4.Select bake function.

5.Bake at 330 degrees F for 15 minutes.

Serving Suggestions: Let cool before serving.

Preparation & Cooking Tips: Use semi-sweet chocolate chips.

72

BLONDIES

Preparation Time: 15 minutes

Cooking Time: 15 minutes

Servings: 4

Ingredients:

•Cooking spray

•6 tablespoons butter, melted

•2 egg yolks

•1 cup brown sugar

•Salt to taste

•1 teaspoon vanilla extract

•1 teaspoon baking powder

•1 cup all-purpose flour

•1 cup butterscotch chips

•½ cup pecans, diced

Method:

1.Spray a small baking pan with oil.

2.In a bowl, mix the butter, egg yolks, brown sugar, salt and vanilla.

3.Stir in the baking powder and flour.

4.Fold in the flour and baking powder.

5.Pour into the pan.

6.Place the pan inside the unit.

7.Select bake function.

8.Bake at 320 degrees F for 15 to 20 minutes.

Serving Suggestions: Let cool before slicing and serving.

Preparation & Cooking Tips: Insert toothpick into the blondie. If it comes out clean, it means that the blondie is fully cooked.

30-DAY MEAL PLAN

Day 1
    Breakfast: Tater Tot Egg Bake
    Lunch: Grilled Steak with Asparagus
    Dinner: Mahi & Salsa
Day 2
    Breakfast: Breakfast Tart
    Lunch: Cheeseburger
    Dinner: Shrimp Tacos
Day 3
    Breakfast: French Toast Sticks
    Lunch: Grilled Steak & Salad
    Dinner: Salmon with Lemon & Dill
Day 4
    Breakfast: Breakfast Casserole
    Lunch: Pot Roast
    Dinner: Lemon Mustard Fish
Day 5
    Breakfast: Quiche
    Lunch: Steak & Potatoes
    Dinner: Shrimp Bang

Day 6
Breakfast: Breakfast Burrito
Lunch: Barbecue Beef Short Ribs
Dinner: Fried Clams
Day 7
Breakfast: Avocado Toast
Lunch: Italian Meatballs
Dinner: Shrimp Tempura
Day 8
Breakfast: Buttermilk Pancake
Lunch: Roast Beef with Chimichurri
Dinner: Garlic Butter Shrimp
Day 9
Breakfast: Cheesy Baked Eggs
Lunch: Garlic Steak with Creamy Horseradish
Dinner: Swordfish Fillet with Salsa
Day 10
Breakfast: Sausage Patties
Lunch: Parmesan Crusted Steak
Dinner: Tuna Burger
Day 11
Breakfast: Tater Tot Egg Bake
Lunch: Grilled Pork Fillet with Veggies
Dinner: Maple Glazed Squash
Day 12
Breakfast: Breakfast Tart
Lunch: Fried Pork Cutlets & Potatoes
Dinner: Veggie Flatbread
Day 13
Breakfast: French Toast Sticks
Lunch: Pork Sandwich
Dinner: Mexican Corn
Day 14
Breakfast: Breakfast Casserole
Lunch: Bacon Wrapped Pork Tenderloin
Dinner: Roasted Potatoes & Asparagus

Day 15
Breakfast: Quiche
Lunch: Sausage & Peppers
Dinner: Lemon Pepper Brussels Sprouts
Day 16
Breakfast: Breakfast Burrito
Lunch: Honey Glazed Ham
Dinner: Balsamic Roasted Tomatoes with Herbs
Day 17
Breakfast: Avocado Toast
Lunch: Bratwursts
Dinner: Squash with Thyme & Sage
Day 18
Breakfast: Buttermilk Pancake
Lunch: Apricot Pork Chops
Dinner: Garlic Carrots
Day 19
Breakfast: Cheesy Baked Eggs
Lunch: Breaded Pork Chops
Dinner: Zucchini Fritters
Day 20
Breakfast: Sausage Patties
Lunch: Pork Tenderloin
Dinner: Buffalo Cauliflower
Day 21
Breakfast: Tater Tot Egg Bake
Lunch: Honey Mustard Chicken
Dinner: Buffalo Cauliflower
Day 22
Breakfast: Breakfast Tart
Lunch: Spicy Ranch Fried Chicken
Dinner: Mahi& Salsa
Day 23
Breakfast: French Toast Sticks
Lunch: Lemon Mustard Chicken
Dinner: Zucchini Fritters

Day 24
Breakfast: Breakfast Casserole
Lunch: Herb-Roasted Chicken
Dinner: Shrimp Tacos

Day 25
Breakfast: Quiche
Lunch: Chicken Teriyaki
Dinner: Garlic Carrots

Day 26
Breakfast: Breakfast Burrito
Lunch: Cajun Chicken
Dinner: Shrimp Bang

Day 27
Breakfast: Avocado Toast
Lunch: Paprika Chicken
Dinner: Squash with Thyme & Sage

Day 28
Breakfast: Buttermilk Pancake
Lunch: Chicken Stuffed with Herbs & Cream Cheese
Dinner: Fried Clams

Day 29
Breakfast: Cheesy Baked Eggs
Lunch: Honey Sriracha Chicken
Dinner: Roasted Potatoes & Asparagus

Day 30
Breakfast: Sausage Patties
Lunch: Barbecue Chicken
Dinner: Swordfish Fillet with Salsa

AFTERWORD

The excitement of being able to cook mouthwatering summer grilled recipes indoors all year round is something that you won't be able to get over with!

But remember, planning is the key to make the most of this opportunity to cook traditional barbecue dishes with the same gorgeous grill marks and distinct summer aroma but without the usual fuss and cleanup.

This book that gives you recipes that you can make with the Ninja Foodie Smart XL Grill is surely a huge help.

With this, you can mix and match the dishes and come up with your favorite pairings for the rest of the year.